UTERINE CANCER DIET

Guide In Managing Symptoms And Improving Their Overall Health.

Charles D. Andersen

Table of Contents

CHAPTER1

What is uterine disease,

Uterine disease, otherwise called endometrial malignant growth, is a sort of disease that starts in the uterus. A woman's uterus is a pear-shaped organ in her pelvis that is important for both menstruation and pregnancy. The most prevalent type of gynecologic cancer affecting women after menopause is uterine cancer. It happens when cells in the coating of the uterus, called the endometrial, begin to develop and duplicate wildly.

The prologue to uterine malignant growth gives an essential comprehension of this sickness. It is essential to understand that uterine cancer is not a single illness but rather a group of various uterine-specific cancers. Endometrial cancer, which begins in the uterine lining, is the most prevalent type. Uterine sarcoma, which develops in the uterine muscle or other tissues, is one of the less common types. It is pivotal to comprehend the gamble factors related with uterine malignant growth, including age, stoutness, hormonal irregular characteristics, and a background marked by specific circumstances like polycystic ovary condition or Lynch disorder.

It is essential to have a basic understanding of uterine cancer for early detection and prevention. Abnormal vaginal bleeding, which can range from spotting to heavy bleeding, is one of the main signs of uterine cancer. Other symptoms include pain in the pelvis, pain during sexual activity, and weight loss that is not explained. It is essential to recognize these symptoms and seek immediate medical attention. Uterine cancer can be detected earlier with regular pelvic exams and pap smears, increasing the likelihood of successful treatment.

CHAPTER2

Types of uterine cancer and the risk factors

All in all, uterine disease is a predominant sort of malignant growth that influences the uterus. Understanding the various types of uterine cancer and the risk factors associated with them is essential. It is essential to recognize the symptoms and undergo regular screenings for prompt treatment and early detection. Individuals can take proactive measures to reduce their risk and maintain their overall health by comprehending the fundamentals of uterine cancer.

A type of cancer that begins in the uterus—the organ where a fetus grows during pregnancy—is called uterine cancer. Because it typically begins in the uterine lining known as the endometrium, it is also referred to as endometrial cancer. Uterine disease is quite possibly of the most widely recognized gynecologic malignant growth and influences ladies, as a rule after menopause. Understanding the fundamentals of uterine cancer, including its causes, symptoms, and risk factors, is essential for students.

Uterine cancer's exact cause is still unknown, but certain factors can make a woman more likely to get it. Hormonal imbalance, particularly an excess of estrogen in comparison to progesterone, is one of the most significant risk factors. Stoutness is one more component that expands the gamble, as fat cells produce estrogen. A family history of ovarian or uterine cancer, age (the risk goes up with age, especially after menopause), and certain medical conditions like diabetes or polycystic ovary syndrome are additional risk factors.

Last but not least, uterine cancer can also be caused by environmental factors. The risk may be exacerbated by exposure to certain chemicals, such as pesticides and cleaning products. Furthermore, radiation treatment focused on the pelvic region, used to treat different sorts of diseases, can likewise expand the gamble of creating uterine malignant growth. When undergoing radiation therapy, it is essential to limit exposure to harmful chemicals and discuss potential risks with healthcare professionals.

CHAPTER3

Symptoms of Uterine cancer's disease.

The side effects of uterine disease can differ, however the most widely recognized sign is unusual vaginal dying, particularly after menopause. Ladies might encounter weighty or delayed periods, draining between periods, or draining after sex. Pain in the pelvis, difficulty urinating, or pain during sexual activity is additional signs. Because early detection and treatment can significantly improve the prognosis, it is essential for women to seek medical attention whenever they experience any of these symptoms.

Students must have a general understanding of uterine cancer in order to be aware of the risks and symptoms of this disease. People can reduce their risk of developing uterine cancer by learning about it and taking the necessary precautions, like keeping a healthy weight and getting regular medical checkups. Moreover, perceiving the side effects and looking for brief clinical consideration can prompt early determination and better treatment results. In the end, raising awareness of uterine cancer can help women's overall health and healthcare.

A type of cancer that affects the uterus—the female reproductive organ where a fetus develops—is known as endometrial cancer. Students must comprehend the causes of uterine cancer in order to raise awareness of the condition and possibly lower their risk of developing it.

The essential driver of uterine malignant growth is hormonal unevenness. Estrogen, a chemical answerable for the development and improvement of the uterus, can in some cases become imbalanced, prompting an excess of the uterine covering. Eventually, this excessive growth may result in cancerous cells. Obesity, diabetes, and polycystic ovary syndrome (PCOS) are all potential contributors to hormonal imbalances. Additionally, prolonged estrogen exposure increases the risk of developing uterine cancer in women who have never been pregnant, began menstruating young, or entered menopause later in life.

One more reason for uterine malignant growth is hereditary transformations. Certain acquired quality transformations, for example, Lynch disorder, can build the gamble of fostering this malignant growth. Lynch disorder is a genetic condition that improves the probability of a few sorts of malignant growths, including uterine disease. People who have a family history of uterine cancer or other cancers that are related should be aware of these genetic factors and talk to a doctor about the right screening and prevention measures

Understanding the reasons for uterine disease can assist understudies with settling on informed decisions to diminish their gamble. Keeping a sound way of life, for example, keeping a solid weight, practicing routinely, and overseeing constant circumstances like diabetes, can assist with directing chemical levels and lessen the gamble of hormonal uneven characters. In addition, genetic counseling and screening should be considered for people who have a family history of uterine cancer in order to catch any inherited mutations early. Lastly, the risk of developing uterine cancer can be further reduced by being aware of potential dangers in the environment and taking the necessary precautions, such as wearing protective gear when handling chemicals. Students can take charge of their own health and well-being by understanding the causes and taking preventative measures.

A type of cancer that begins in the uterine lining is called uterine cancer, or endometrial cancer. The most prevalent form of cancer affecting the female reproductive system is this one. For early detection and prompt treatment, it is essential to comprehend uterine cancer symptoms.

Abnormal vaginal bleeding is one of the most common symptoms of uterine cancer. This can appear as spotting between feminine periods, draining after menopause, or curiously weighty or delayed periods. Women may also experience persistent or intermittent pelvic pain or discomfort. Pain during sexual activity is another possible symptom. Furthermore, a few ladies might see changes in their urinary or gut propensities, like successive pee or clogging.

It's critical to keep in mind that these symptoms can also be brought on by other conditions, and just because a person has one or more of them doesn't mean they have uterine cancer. Nonetheless, in the event that any of these side effects persevere or decline, counseling a medical services proficient for additional evaluation is pivotal. Uterine cancer can be detected early and treated more effectively, leading to better outcomes. Gynecological screenings and exams, like Pap smears and pelvic exams, should be done on a regular basis to keep an eye on and find any problems with the uterus.

In conclusion, women's health depends on knowing about

uterine cancer symptoms. Individuals who are aware of changes in their urinary or bowel habits, abnormal vaginal bleeding, pelvic pain, pain during sexual activity, and other symptoms can seek immediate medical attention. It is critical to recollect that these side effects can be brought about by different variables, however it is in every case better to decide in favor alert and counsel a medical services proficient for an exhaustive assessment. Early identification and therapy can altogether work on the anticipation for uterine disease patients

. A type of cancer known as uterine cancer affects the uterus, the female reproductive organ that is in charge of supporting and feeding a developing fetus. This disease ordinarily starts in the coating of the uterus, called the endometrium, and is known as endometrial malignant growth. Patients and their families must have a solid

CHAPTER4

Uterine cancer's diagnosis
prevention and treatment

Understanding of uterine cancer's diagnosis and treatment options in order to make educated decisions and successfully navigate the recovery process.

A thorough medical history and physical examination typically serve as the foundation for a uterine cancer diagnosis. To confirm the diagnosis of uterine cancer, additional tests may be ordered if it is suspected. These tests might incorporate imaging concentrates, for example, ultrasounds, CT sweeps, or X-rays to assess the size and degree of the disease. Moreover, a biopsy is frequently performed to get an example of the uterine tissue for investigation under a magnifying lens. This biopsy should be possible through an insignificantly obtrusive method called hysteroscopy or by eliminating a little piece of tissue during a widening and curettage (D&C) system.

The healthcare team will create an individual treatment plan based on the patient's overall health as well as the stage and grade of the cancer once the diagnosis of uterine cancer has been confirmed. Surgery, radiation therapy, chemotherapy, or a combination of these treatments may be used to treat uterine cancer. Medical procedure is in many cases the essential therapy for beginning phase uterine disease and may include eliminating the uterus (hysterectomy) alongside encompassing tissues and lymph hubs. Women who want to keep their ability to have children may occasionally have the option of having fertility-sparing surgery. High-energy beams are used in radiation therapy to kill cancer cells, while drugs are used in chemotherapy to kill cancer cells all over the body.

All in all, the determination and therapy of uterine disease require a complete methodology that includes different clinical trials and strategies. Through cautious assessment and examination, medical services experts can precisely analyze uterine malignant growth and decide the most fitting therapy plan for every patient. It is fundamental for patients to work intimately with their medical services group, get clarification on some things, and look for help from friends and family all through their excursion to oversee and defeat uterine disease actually.

Cancer prevention and treatment both rely heavily on nutrition. Studies have demonstrated the way that a sound eating routine and way of life can diminish the gamble of creating disease. A diet high in fruits, vegetables, whole grains, and lean proteins can help you maintain a healthy weight and supply the body's immune system with essential nutrients. On the other hand, eating a diet that is high in processed and red meat, refined sugar, and unhealthy fats can make it more likely that you will get cancer

During malignant growth treatment, sustenance is pivotal for keeping up with strength and endurance. Disease patients frequently experience incidental effects like queasiness, heaving, and loss of craving, which can prompt lack of healthy sustenance. A well-balanced diet consisting of smaller, more frequent meals can support the body's healing process and reduce these side effects. It is likewise vital to remain hydrated and to talk with an enlisted dietitian to make a customized sustenance plan.

Although nutrition cannot treat cancer, it can support the body's ability to combat the disease. A solid eating regimen can assist with lessening irritation, support sound cell development, and lift the resistant framework. Furthermore, certain food sources have been displayed to have disease battling properties, for example, cruciferous vegetables like broccoli and kale, which contain intensifies that can assist with forestalling disease cell development. Including a variety of fruits and vegetables in your diet and avoiding processed and high-fat foods can support overall health and reduce the risk of cancer.

The prevention of cancer is largely dependent on diet. Consuming a sound, adjusted diet that is wealthy in natural products, vegetables, entire grains, and incline proteins can assist with diminishing the gamble of creating disease. The American Malignant growth Society suggests filling your plate with various bright products of the soil, as they contain nutrients, minerals, and cancer prevention agents that can assist with shielding cells from harm that can prompt disease. Limiting processed and red meat consumption, as well as sugar-laden beverages and snacks, can also lower cancer risk.

The uterus, the female reproductive organ that is responsible for menstruation and pregnancy, is the site of uterine cancer. For effective treatment and early detection of uterine cancer, it is essential to recognize and manage its symptoms. Abnormal vaginal bleeding, pelvic pain, difficulty urinating, and pain during sexual activity are all common signs of uterine cancer. People genuinely should know about these side effects and immediately talk with a medical services proficient in the event that they experience any of them. The likelihood of a successful treatment and recovery greatly increases when uterine cancer is detected early.

Uterine cancer treatment options include surgery, radiation therapy, and chemotherapy, in addition to identifying symptoms. Uterine cancer is typically treated primarily through surgery, which involves the removal of the uterus and the tissues that surround it. Radiation treatment utilizes high-energy shafts to kill disease cells and is much of the time utilized in mix with a medical procedure to focus on any leftover malignant growth cells. Chemotherapy, on the other hand, uses drugs to kill cancer cells all over the body. It is usually used to stop a recurrence or treat advanced cases. Individuals who have been diagnosed with uterine cancer must collaborate closely with their healthcare team to select the most effective treatment strategy based on their particular condition and requirements.

CHAPTER5

How to Maintain a healthy diets

Besides, keeping a sound load through legitimate nourishment and standard activity can likewise assist with forestalling disease. The American Cancer Society says that being overweight or obese can make you more likely to get breast, colon, and pancreatic cancer, among other types. Maintaining a healthy weight and lowering the risk of cancer can both be aided by following a diet low in processed foods and high in fiber.

Furthermore, standard activity can assist with diminishing irritation in the body, which can likewise bring down the gamble of disease.

All in all, the significance of nourishment in disease counteraction couldn't possibly be more significant. People can reduce their risk of developing cancer by eating a diet high in fruits, vegetables, whole grains, and lean proteins and avoiding processed and red meat, as well as sugary snacks and beverages. Moreover, keeping a solid load through legitimate nourishment and ordinary activity can likewise assist with forestalling disease. By making little, maintainable changes to their eating regimen and way of life, people can make proactive strides towards decreasing their gamble of malignant growth and advancing generally speaking wellbeing and health.

Sustenance assumes a pivotal part in the therapy of disease patients. A very much arranged diet can assist patients with dealing with the symptoms of disease treatment and work on their general personal satisfaction. Common side effects of chemotherapy or radiation therapy include fatigue, nausea, and vomiting. Patients can help maintain their weight, strengthen their immune system, and lower their risk of infection by eating a diet that is high in protein, calories, and essential nutrients.

In order to avoid malnutrition, which can make it harder for cancer patients to tolerate treatment and increase their risk of complications, they must also be careful about what they eat. An eating routine that incorporates different natural products, vegetables, entire grains, lean proteins, and solid fats can give the supplements expected to the body to appropriately work. In addition, some cancer treatments may make osteoporosis more likely, so it's important to get enough calcium and vitamin D to keep your bones healthy.

A healthy diet can also assist cancer patients in managing their symptoms and improving their overall health. Constipation, a common side effect of treating cancer, can be alleviated by eating a diet high in fiber. Moreover, devouring food varieties that are high in cell reinforcements, like berries, green verdant vegetables, and nuts, can assist with decreasing aggravation and oxidative pressure in the body.

Patients can focus on their recovery and feel more at ease by managing symptoms like pain, nausea, and fatigue.

In conclusion, cancer treatment relies heavily on nutrition. Eating a very much arranged diet can assist patients with dealing with the symptoms of treatment, forestall hunger, and further develop their general prosperity. A registered dietitian should be consulted by cancer patients to develop an individual nutrition plan that meets their specific requirements and preferences. Cancer patients can improve their health and increase their chances of a full recovery by eating a well-balanced diet high in essential nutrients.

Uterine disease is a kind of malignant growth that creates in the uterus, the female regenerative organ where fetal improvement happens. The disease is brought about by strange development of cells in the coating of the uterus, and it tends to be made do with legitimate nourishment. A healthy diet can help the body's immune system and reduce inflammation, two important aspects of disease management.

Consuming a diet that is high in fruits and vegetables is one of the most important nutrition strategies for managing uterine cancer. Products of the soil are stacked with cancer prevention agents, which help to lessen irritation and safeguard cells from harm. The absolute best foods grown from the ground to remember for your eating routine incorporate salad greens, berries, broccoli, and carrots. These food sources are likewise high in fiber, which can assist with advancing sound processing and forestall stoppage, a typical symptom of malignant growth treatment.

Lean proteins like chicken, fish, and legumes are also important to eat in addition to fruits and vegetables. Protein is essential for the body's ability to build new cells and repair damaged tissues, both of which are necessary for managing uterine cancer. Also important is to avoid processed and sugary foods because they can cause inflammation and may make you more likely to have other health issues. You can contribute to the management of uterine cancer and enhance your overall health and well-being by eating a nutritious diet that is high in whole foods.

In both the treatment and prevention of cancer, nutrition plays an essential role. People who have cancer or are at risk of developing it need to eat a healthy diet. The objective of carrying out a nutritious eating routine is to advance generally wellbeing and prosperity, work on the resistant framework, and lessen the gamble of disease. A sound eating routine can likewise assist with overseeing malignant growth side effects and symptoms of disease medicines, like weakness, sickness, and weight reduction.

A nutritious eating regimen for malignant growth counteraction and the board incorporates various organic products, vegetables, entire grains, lean proteins, and sound fats. It is prescribed to restrict the admission of handled food sources and sweet beverages, as they can expand the gamble of malignant growth. It is additionally critical to remain hydrated by drinking a lot of water and keeping away from liquor. Keeping a solid load through a fair eating routine and customary activity can likewise assist with diminishing the gamble of malignant growth.

Carrying out a nutritious eating routine can be testing, particularly for malignant growth patients who might encounter changes in hunger and taste. Working with an enlisted dietitian can assist with fostering a customized sustenance plan that addresses individual issues and inclinations. To ensure adequate nutrient intake, nutritional supplements like protein powders and vitamins may also be suggested. In addition, it can be easier to stick to a healthy diet when family members and caregivers participate in meal planning and preparation.

In conclusion, a healthy diet is a crucial component of cancer prevention and treatment. A healthy diet can help manage symptoms and side effects of cancer treatments as well as lower the risk of developing the disease. Working with an enrolled dietitian and including relatives and guardians can assist with making it more straightforward to keep a sound eating regimen. By focusing on nourishment, people can play a functioning job in their wellbeing and prosperity.

Maintaining a well-balanced and nutritious diet necessitates the creation of a healthy meal plan. It includes cautiously choosing food sources and getting ready dinners that meet the body's wholesome necessities. People can improve their overall health and well-being by understanding the fundamentals of creating a healthy meal plan.

CHAPTER6

How to make a good feast plan,

With regards to making a good feast plan, it is vital to initially grasp the idea of adjusted sustenance. This implies consolidating an assortment of nutrition classes in your dinners to guarantee that you are getting every one of the important supplements. These nutrition classes ordinarily incorporate foods grown from the ground, entire grains, lean proteins, and sound fats. Every one of these nutrition types assumes a fundamental part in furnishing the body with fundamental nutrients, minerals, and energy.

As well as considering the different nutrition classes, it is significant to focus on segment sizes and dinner timing. In order to control how many calories you consume and keep a healthy weight, portion control is essential. Instead of eating a lot all at once, it's better to eat smaller, more balanced meals throughout the day. This assists with keeping energy levels stable and forestalls gorging. Additionally, it is essential to schedule meals at regular intervals to prevent excessive hunger or cravings and provide the body with energy throughout the day.

Last but not least, making meals enjoyable requires including a variety of flavors and textures in a healthy meal plan. Explore different avenues regarding various flavors, spices, and flavors to upgrade the flavor of dishes without depending on undesirable added substances like extreme salt or sugar. Also, try to include both cooked and raw foods to get the most nutrients and different textures. Individuals can develop a balanced, healthy meal plan that supports their overall health and well-being by adhering to these guidelines.

A quality dinner plan is critical for keeping up with great wellbeing and generally speaking prosperity. In order for us to make well-informed decisions regarding our diet, it is essential to comprehend the significance of a healthy meal plan. A quality dinner, first and foremost, plan guarantees that our body gets every one of the important supplements it requirements to appropriately work. By including different natural products, vegetables, entire grains, lean proteins, and solid fats in our dinners, we can give our body the fundamental nutrients, minerals, and cell reinforcements it expects for ideal wellbeing.

Furthermore, a good dinner plan can assist with forestalling the beginning of persistent infections like stoutness, diabetes, and coronary illness. By keeping away from inordinate utilization of handled food sources, sweet drinks, and unfortunate fats, we can diminish the gamble of fostering these circumstances. An even feast plan that incorporates suitable piece sizes and an emphasis on supplement thick food sources can likewise assist with keeping a sound weight, which is helpful for in general wellbeing.

Finally, a good dinner plan can decidedly influence our energy levels and temperament. At the point when we fuel our body with nutritious food varieties, we give it the important fuel to really work. We may experience increased alertness and focus throughout the day as a result of this. Additionally, certain foods, such as those high in B vitamins and omega-3 fatty acids, have been shown to improve mood. By integrating these food varieties into our dinner plan, we can uphold our psychological prosperity and possibly diminish the gamble of temperament issues.

In conclusion, in order to make well-informed choices regarding our diet, it is essential to comprehend the significance of a healthy meal plan. An even dinner plan guarantees that our body gets the essential supplements, forestalls ongoing infections, and can emphatically influence our energy levels and temperament. We can make a healthy meal plan that helps us feel and look our best by putting nutrient-dense foods first and not eating too many unhealthy options.

For the purpose of preserving one's general health and preventing a variety of diseases, developing a nutritious meal plan is essential. When creating a meal plan, it is essential to take into account a diet that is well-balanced and contains all of the essential nutrients. A quality dinner plan ought to comprise of different natural products, vegetables, entire grains, lean proteins, and solid fats. These foods contain essential vitamins, minerals, and antioxidants that help maintain good health and lower the risk of chronic conditions like diabetes, certain types of cancer, and heart disease.

The uterus, the female reproductive organ that is responsible for menstruation and pregnancy, is the site of uterine cancer. For effective treatment and early detection of uterine cancer, it is essential to recognize and manage its symptoms. Abnormal vaginal bleeding, pelvic pain, difficulty urinating, and pain during sexual activity are all common signs of uterine cancer. People genuinely should know about these side effects and immediately talk with a medical services proficient in the event that they experience any of them. The likelihood of a successful treatment and recovery greatly increases when uterine cancer is detected early.

All in all, making a quality dinner plan is pivotal for keeping up with great wellbeing and diminishing the gamble of different ailments, including uterine malignant growth. Healthy fats, whole grains, lean proteins, and a variety of fruits and vegetables are all part of a well-balanced diet that supports overall health. Identifying and managing symptoms is essential for early detection and effective treatment of uterine cancer. People really should know about the normal side effects of uterine disease and talk with a medical care proficient on the off chance that they experience any of them. People with uterine cancer can also manage their condition and increase their chances of a successful treatment and recovery by working closely with a healthcare team and understanding the various treatment options.

A healthy meal plan is important for your overall health, but it's even more important when you're dealing with a health problem like uterine cancer. Modifying a feast plan for uterine malignant growth the executives includes integrating explicit food sources that can uphold the body's mending and give the vital supplements. A healthy meal plan for managing uterine cancer is built on whole grains, vegetables, lean proteins, and healthy fats.

Entire grains are a phenomenal wellspring of dietary fiber, which supports processing and keeps a solid weight. Integrating entire grains, for example, quinoa, earthy colored rice, and entire wheat bread can give fundamental supplements and energy while decreasing the gamble of weight gain. Leafy foods are plentiful in cell reinforcements, nutrients, and minerals, which can uphold the safe framework and help battle against malignant growth cells. A meal plan can ensure that a wide range of nutrients are consumed by including a variety of colorful fruits and vegetables.

Lean proteins are critical for building and fixing tissues, particularly during disease treatment. Lean protein sources like fish without the skin, tofu, legumes, and poultry can provide the necessary amino acids without adding too many unhealthy fats. Avocados, nuts, and olive oil are all good sources of healthy fats, which are important for brain health and reducing inflammation. Remembering these fats for control can assist with keeping up with generally speaking wellbeing and give a feeling of satiety.

Individual dietary restrictions or sensitivities should also be taken into account in a individualized meal plan for the management of uterine cancer. It is critical to talk with a medical services proficient or an enrolled dietitian to make a customized dinner plan that considers a particular necessities or concerns. Additionally, it is essential for overall health and well-being to drink plenty of water and avoid sugary beverages to stay hydrated. Individuals can support their bodies in managing uterine cancer and promote overall health and well-being by customizing a meal plan with these essential components. Making a good dinner plan is fundamental for keeping a reasonable eating regimen and accomplishing generally prosperity. One significant part of effective feast arranging is understanding tips and apparatuses that can assist people with accomplishing their dietary objectives. When planning meals, it's helpful to set goals that are within your reach. It's critical to take into account personal preferences, time constraints, and budgetary constraints. People are more likely to adhere to their diet and succeed in their dietary endeavors if they set attainable goals.

Another dinner plan that can be useful for uterine malignant growth anticipation is the plant-based diet. Fruits, vegetables, whole grains, legumes, nuts, and other plant-based foods are the primary staples of this diet.

Additionally, it restricts or eliminates animal products like eggs, dairy, and meat. It has been demonstrated that this kind of diet lowers the risk of several kinds of cancer, including uterine cancer. Additionally, plant-based diets frequently have fewer calories and can aid in weight loss, which is crucial for lowering uterine cancer risk.

CHAPTER7

Recipes for meal planning.

Using a variety of resources to find recipes and meal ideas is another helpful tool for meal planning. Sites, cookbooks, and, surprisingly, versatile applications can give an abundance of motivation to making solid and flavorful feasts. These assets frequently offer many recipes custom fitted to various dietary requirements and inclinations. By investigating various sources, people can find intriguing feast choices, guaranteeing that their dinner plan stays fascinating and agreeable.

Ultimately, it is significant to integrate dinner preparing into the feast arranging process. Preparing and portioning meals ahead of time, or meal prepping, makes it simpler to adhere to a meal plan throughout the week. People can save time and avoid the temptation to eat unhealthy foods by planning and preparing their meals ahead of time each week. Feast preparing can likewise assist with segment control, as pre-divided dinners can forestall indulging. By carrying out these tips and using these devices, people can make a fruitful and compelling feast plan for keeping a sound way of life.

Uterine malignant growth is a sort of disease that influences the uterus, the female regenerative organ liable for lodging and supporting a creating embryo during pregnancy. Uterine cancer is the fourth most common cancer in women, with over 60,000 new cases diagnosed annually, according to the American Cancer Society. Although the exact cause of uterine cancer is unknown, obesity, a high-fat diet, and a sedentary lifestyle are three lifestyle factors that can increase a woman's risk of developing this disease. On the other hand, there are a number of recipes and meal plans that can assist in controlling or preventing uterine cancer.

One recipe that is especially gainful for uterine malignant growth counteraction is the Mediterranean eating regimen. Whole grains, fruits, and lean protein sources like fish and poultry are abundant in this diet. While limiting saturated and trans fats, it also places an emphasis on healthy fats like olive oil and nuts. Studies have shown that ladies who follow a Mediterranean eating routine have a lower hazard of creating uterine malignant growth, as well as different kinds of disease and ongoing infections.

Last but not least, it's important to remember that drinking less alcohol can also help prevent uterine cancer. Women who drink more than one alcoholic beverage per day are more likely to develop uterine cancer, according to research. Hence, integrating non-cocktails into your feast plans, like water, tea, or shimmering water, can be a basic yet viable method for lessening your gamble of this sickness. You can help lower your risk of uterine cancer and improve your overall health and wellness by eating a well-balanced diet.

Healthy eating is important for everyone, but it's especially important for people who are at risk for uterine cancer and have to deal with it. A solid eating regimen can assist with diminishing the gamble of creating disease, as well as help to oversee side effects and results of malignant growth treatment. To present good dieting for uterine disease counteraction and the executives, it is vital to comprehend what kinds of food varieties are helpful and what ought to be stayed away from.

One of the main parts of a sound eating routine for uterine disease counteraction and the board is the utilization of leafy foods. These food varieties are plentiful in nutrients, minerals, and cell reinforcements that can assist with supporting the resistant framework, battle aggravation, and decrease the gamble of malignant growth. A few instances of sound products of the soil incorporate salad greens, berries, citrus natural products, and cruciferous vegetables like broccoli and cauliflower.

Lean protein sources are another important part of a healthy diet for preventing and treating uterine cancer. Protein is fundamental for keeping up with bulk and strength, and furthermore assists with keeping you feeling full and fulfilled. A few instances of sound protein sources incorporate lean meats like chicken and fish, as well as plant-based choices like beans, lentils, and tofu.

Last but not least, it's important to limit or avoid certain foods that can make symptoms worse or raise the risk of uterine cancer. This incorporates handled food sources, sweet beverages, and food varieties high in soaked and trans fats. As excessive alcohol consumption has been linked to an increased risk of uterine cancer, it should also be consumed in moderation. By making these solid dietary changes, people can assist with diminishing their gamble of uterine malignant growth and work on their general wellbeing and prosperity

Uterine malignant growth is a sort of disease that emerges in the uterus, the female conceptive organ liable for monthly cycle and pregnancy. Uterine cancer's exact cause is unknown, but certain risk factors like obesity, diabetes, and hormonal imbalances can make it more likely to happen. On the other hand, uterine cancer can be prevented or treated with the help of a healthy diet that includes lean proteins, whole grains, fruits, and vegetables. In this regard, a meal plan for preventing or treating uterine cancer can include a number of delicious and healthy recipes.

One such recipe is quinoa salad with simmered vegetables. Quinoa is a whole grain that is high in protein and fiber, making it a great option for people who want to keep their weight in a healthy range. Antioxidants in roasted vegetables like sweet potatoes, zucchini, and peppers help to prevent cell damage and lower the risk of cancer. To make this recipe, cook quinoa as per bundle guidelines and meal vegetables in the broiler until delicate. Join quinoa and vegetables in a bowl and dress with a combination of olive oil, lemon juice, and spices like parsley and thyme.

Salmon with roasted asparagus and brown rice is another delicious and healthy recipe for preventing or treating uterine cancer. Omega-3 fatty acids, which have been shown to lower cancer risk and reduce inflammation, are abundant in salmon, a fatty fish. Asparagus is a low-calorie vegetable that is high in fiber and folate, a supplement that is fundamental for sound cell development. As a whole grain with a low glycemic index and a high fiber content, brown rice is an excellent option for diabetics. Roast asparagus until tender and bake salmon fillets in the oven for this recipe. Present with earthy colored rice and a crush of lemon juice.

Fresh fruit salad with Greek yogurt is a delicious and healthy dessert option for uterine cancer prevention or treatment. Greek yogurt is a dairy product high in protein and low in sugar and fat, making it a healthy alternative to ice cream and other traditional desserts. Antioxidants and vitamins found in fresh fruits like mango, kiwi, and berries can help prevent cancer. Chop up a variety of fresh fruits, combine them with Greek yogurt and honey, and then serve. Serve chilled.

In conclusion, uterine cancer can be prevented or treated with a healthy diet that includes lean proteins, whole grains, fruits, and vegetables. A meal plan for preventing or treating uterine cancer can include a number of delicious and healthy recipes. Salmon with roasted asparagus and brown rice, quinoa salad with roasted vegetables, and fresh fruit salad with Greek yogurt are among these recipes. People can reduce their risk of developing uterine cancer and improve their overall health and well-being by incorporating these recipes into a meal plan.

A healthy diet is one of the best ways to prevent or treat uterine cancer. Feast arranging is a brilliant technique to guarantee you are getting the supplements your body needs to keep up with ideal wellbeing. A very much arranged feast can likewise assist you with keeping a solid weight, which is one more urgent consider decreasing your gamble of uterine disease.

Focus on including foods high in fiber, vitamins, and minerals when planning your meals. Food sources, for example, cruciferous vegetables like broccoli, cabbage, and kale, vegetables, entire grains, and organic products are fantastic decisions. Additionally, these foods have anti-inflammatory properties that may assist in lowering your risk of developing uterine cancer and reducing inflammation.

It is likewise vital for limit your admission of red and handled meats, sweet food varieties, and refined sugars. These food varieties have been connected to an expanded gamble of malignant growth, including uterine disease. All things considered, select lean proteins like chicken, fish, and plant-based proteins like beans and lentils. You can lower your risk of uterine cancer and improve your overall health by incorporating these meal planning strategies.

THE   END